Myositis

A Beginner's 3-Step Guide to Managing
Autoimmune Disorders including
Dermatomyositis and Polymyositis Through
Diet, with Sample Curated Recipes

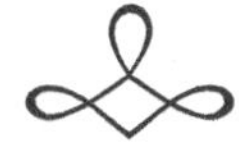

PATRICK MARSHWELL

Disclaimer

By reading this disclaimer, you are accepting the terms of the disclaimer in full. If you disagree with this disclaimer, please do not use this website.

All of the content within this website is provided for informational and educational purposes only, and should not be accepted as independent medical or other professional advice. The author of these articles is not a doctor, physician, nurse, mental health provider, or registered nutritionist/dietician. Therefore, using and reading any of the content on this website does not establish any form of a physician-patient relationship.

Always consult with a physician or another qualified health provider with any issues or questions you might have regarding any sort of medical condition. Do not ever disregard any qualified professional medical advice or delay seeking that advice because of anything you have read in this guide. The information in this guide is not intended to be any sort of medical advice and should not be used in lieu of any medical advice by a licensed and qualified medical professional.

The information on this website has been compiled from a variety of known sources. However, the author cannot attest

rights to use the images through license agreements with third-party stock image companies.

Introduction

Myositis is a general term for a group of rare autoimmune diseases that cause inflammation of the muscles. This inflammation can lead to pain, swelling, and difficulty in moving. The cause of myositis is unknown, but it is thought to be related to an overactive immune system.

There are several different types of myositis, each with its own set of symptoms. The most common type, dermatomyositis, causes a distinctive rash in addition to muscle weakness and inflammation. Inclusion body myositis typically affects older adults and causes slowly progressive muscle weakness. Polymyositis can affect people of any age and often leads to fatigue and difficulty swallowing.

While there is no cure for myositis, early diagnosis and treatment are important for preventing serious complications. Treatment typically involves a combination of medications, physical therapy, and lifestyle changes. A healthy diet is an important part of managing myositis and can help reduce inflammation, improve muscle function, and boost overall health.

In some cases, myositis may go into remission for extended periods. With proper care, people with myositis can lead active and fulfilling lives.

In this beginner's guide, we'll discuss the following in detail:

- What causes myositis?
- What are the three common types of myositis?
- What are the risk factors for myositis?
- What are the complications of myositis?
- How is myositis diagnosed?
- How is myositis treated?
- A potential 3-step plan for managing myositis.
- Managing myositis through diet and nutrition.
- Living with myositis.

Table of Contents

WHAT CAUSES MYOSITIS?

Many different conditions fall under the umbrella of myositis, and the exact cause of each one is not yet known. However, it is believed that myositis occurs when the immune system mistakes healthy cells for foreign invaders and attacks them. This can occur in response to a viral or bacterial infection, or even in the absence of any known trigger. In some cases, myositis may be caused by medications or other substances that interfere with the normal functioning of the immune system.

Whatever its cause, myositis results in inflammation and damage to muscle tissue, which can lead to a wide range of symptoms. These may include muscle weakness, fatigue, joint pain, and difficulty swallowing or breathing. If you experience any of these symptoms, be sure to see a doctor for a proper diagnosis. With treatment, it is often possible to manage myositis and reduce its symptoms.

WHAT ARE THE 3 COMMON TYPES OF MYOSITIS?

Myositis is a rare autoimmune disease that causes inflammation of the muscles. There are three common types of myositis: dermatomyositis, polymyositis, and inclusion body myositis.

1. Dermatomyositis

Dermatomyositis is a rare autoimmune disease that causes inflammation and damage to the muscles. It is the most common type of myositis, and it affects both men and women equally.

This disease most commonly affects adults between the ages of 40 and 60.

Symptoms of dermatomyositis include muscle weakness, fatigue, difficulty breathing, and a rash on the face and chest. The cause of dermatomyositis is unknown, but it is believed to be caused by a combination of genetic and environmental factors. There is no cure for dermatomyositis, but treatment options include medications to suppress the immune system, physical therapy, and in some cases, surgery.

Dermatomyositis Symptoms

<u>Rashes:</u> The most common symptom of dermatomyositis is a rash, which often appears on the face, neck, and chest. The rash is often accompanied by itching and burning.

<u>Muscle weakness:</u> The most common symptom of dermatomyositis is muscle weakness, which can lead to difficulty swallowing and breathing in some cases. Muscle weakness is usually symmetrical, meaning that it affects both sides of the body equally.

<u>Fatigue:</u> Another common symptom of dermatomyositis is fatigue. This can be caused by some factors, including inflammation, muscle weakness, and anemia. The fatigue associated with dermatomyositis can be extreme, and it may interfere with a person's ability to perform daily activities. In some cases, people with dermatomyositis may need to be hospitalized due to the severity of their fatigue.

<u>Joint pain:</u> Joint pain can range from mild stiffness to severe discomfort that limits a person's ability to move. The joints most often affected are those in the hands, wrists, elbows, shoulders, and hips. The pain is typically worse in the morning and improves with activity during the day. It may also be accompanied by swelling, warmth, and redness.

If left untreated, joint pain can lead to joint damage and deformity. Treatment for dermatomyositis-related joint pain typically includes a combination of medication and physical therapy. In some cases, surgery may also be necessary.

While there is no cure for dermatomyositis, treatment can help to reduce symptoms and improve quality of life. Treatment typically involves corticosteroids and immunosuppressants.

2. Polymyositis

Polymyositis is a kind of myositis that affects the muscles and is more severe than dermatomyositis. It is more frequent in those over the age of 50, particularly women, and it is more prevalent in women than in males.

In contrast to dermatomyositis, polymyositis does not manifest itself through the development of rashes. Polymyositis symptoms, on the other hand, can be just as incapacitating as the disease itself. These symptoms include weakness in the muscles, exhaustion, discomfort in the joints, and difficulty swallowing.

3. Inclusion Body Myositis

Myositis can come in a few different forms, but the most severe and unusual one is called inclusion body myositis. It typically affects individuals who are over the age of 50, and males are more likely to be diagnosed with it than women are. Inclusion body myositis is characterized by symptoms that proceed at a considerably more glacial pace than those of the first two forms of myositis.

Inclusion body myositis is a type of myositis that causes inflammation in the muscles as well as damage to the nervous system. While the symptoms of inclusion-body myositis are closely similar to those of the first two types of myositis, the primary difference is that inclusion-body myositis causes damage to the nervous system. This can result in difficulties with walking, balancing, and coordinating movements. People who have inclusion body myositis may, at times, find themselves in need of the assistance of a wheelchair.

WHAT ARE THE RISK FACTORS FOR MYOSITIS?

While the exact cause of myositis is unknown, several risk factors have been identified. These include:

Age: One risk factor for myositis is age. Myositis is most common in adults over the age of 50. This is because as people age, they are more likely to experience a decrease in muscle mass and strength. Additionally, the immune system weakens with age, making it less able to fight off infection. As a result, older adults are more susceptible to developing myositis.

Gender: Women are more likely to develop myositis than men except for inclusion body myositis which is more common in men than women. This may be due to hormonal differences, as estrogen has been shown to play a role in modulating the immune response. Additionally, certain autoimmune diseases are more common in women, and these diseases often share common risk factors with myositis.

Family history: One risk factor for myositis is family history. If you have a close relative, such as a parent or sibling, who has myositis, you're more likely to develop the condition. However, it's important to keep in mind that having a family member with myositis doesn't guarantee that you'll develop the

disorder. Most people with myositis don't have a family history
of the condition.

WHAT ARE THE COMPLICATIONS OF MYOSITIS?

Myositis is a condition that can lead to several complications if left untreated. These complications can include inflammation of the muscles, muscle weakness, and even rhabdomyolysis, which is a potentially fatal condition caused by the breakdown of muscle tissue.

Rhabdomyolysis: Rhabdomyolysis occurs when muscle cells are destroyed and release their contents into the bloodstream. This can cause a variety of problems, including kidney damage, electrolyte imbalances, and even heart failure.

Inflammation of the heart: Heart inflammation is a rare complication of myositis, and can occur in any type of myositis. While the exact cause is unknown, it is thought to be related to an autoimmune reaction. Symptoms of heart inflammation include chest pain, shortness of breath, fatigue, and irregular heartbeat. In severe cases, heart inflammation can lead to congestive heart failure.

Pulmonary complications: Complications of myositis can include pulmonary complications, which refer to problems with the lungs. Pulmonary complications can range from mild to life-threatening, and they are the most common cause of death in people with myositis.

The most common pulmonary complication is interstitial lung disease (ILD), which is a chronic inflammation of the tissues that surround the air sacs in the lungs. ILD can cause shortness of breath, coughing, and fatigue. In severe cases, it can lead to respiratory failure.

Some people with myositis also develop bronchiolitis obliterans, which is a scarring of the small airways in the lungs. Bronchiolitis obliterans can cause shortness of breath, wheezing, and coughing.

Kidney problems: Kidney problems are a potential complication associated with myositis. That's because the kidneys play an important role in filtering toxins from the bloodstream. When myositis results in inflammation of the muscles, it can also lead to kidney damage. In some cases, this can cause kidney failure.

Symptoms of kidney problems include fatigue, nausea, and decreased urination. If you experience any of these symptoms, it's important to see a doctor right away. Kidney problems can be serious, and early diagnosis and treatment are essential to preventing long-term damage.

Skin problems: Myositis is connected with several skin problems, one of the most prevalent of which is cutaneous vasculitis. Inflammation of the blood vessels is the primary symptom of this condition, which can also present as redness, itching, and discomfort. It is also possible for cutaneous vasculitis to result in ulceration, and more severe situations, necrosis. Cutaneous vasculitis more frequently affects smaller blood vessels, however, there have been reports of it affecting larger blood vessels as well.

Cases of cutaneous vasculitis linked with myositis are often minor, and the disease frequently clears up following effective treatment of the myositis that lies beneath the skin. However, in certain cases, cutaneous vasculitis may continue to manifest itself even after the myositis has been brought under control, and it may be necessary to take further steps to treat the skin disease.

It is important for people who have been diagnosed with myositis to seek treatment as soon as possible to help prevent these complications from occurring.

HOW IS MYOSITIS DIAGNOSED?

Visit a medical professional as soon as you can if you or a member of your family has any reason to think that you or they have myositis. In the absence of treatment, myositis is a severe illness that has the risk of developing consequences that might be fatal.

A diagnosis of myositis is often arrived at after a patient has had a series of diagnostic procedures, including a physical exam, imaging tests, blood tests, and muscle biopsies.

Physical exam: A healthcare professional can diagnose myositis through a physical examination. One common sign of myositis is muscle weakness. The healthcare professional will test the strength of the muscles by asking the person to resist pressure or by observing the range of motion of the joints. Another sign of myositis is muscle inflammation. The healthcare professional will look for tenderness, redness, and swelling in the muscles.

Blood tests: Blood tests are often used to diagnose myositis. There are a few different types of blood tests that can be ordered, and each type of test can provide important information about the presence and severity of myositis. For example, a blood test called a creatine kinase test can be used to measure levels of a protein that is released when muscle cells are damaged. This test can help to confirm the diagnosis of myositis, as well as to determine how much muscle damage has occurred.

Blood tests can also be used to measure levels of inflammation, which can help to identify the cause of myositis. In some cases, a blood test may be the only test that is needed to diagnose myositis. However, in other cases, additional testing may be required to confirm the diagnosis.

Muscle biopsy: One way to diagnose myositis is through a muscle biopsy. In this procedure, a small sample of muscle tissue is removed and examined for inflammation. A muscle biopsy can be performed as an outpatient procedure, and it is generally safe and well-tolerated.

The main risk of a muscle biopsy is bleeding from the incision site. However, this complication is rare and can usually be controlled with a pressure dressing. Overall, a muscle biopsy is an effective way to diagnose myositis and should be considered in patients who have suggestive symptoms. With early diagnosis, patients can begin treatment and improve their prognosis.

Imaging tests: While there are a variety of blood tests and biopsies that can be used to diagnose myositis, imaging tests such as MRI and CT scans can also be helpful. These tests can provide detailed information about the location and extent of muscle inflammation. In some cases, they may also reveal other abnormalities, such as calcium deposits in the muscles.

Imaging tests are often used in conjunction with other diagnostic tools to arrive at a final diagnosis.

EMG testing: The most common way of diagnosing myositis is through EMG testing. This is a test where electrical impulses are sent through the muscles to determine if they are functioning properly. Myositis can cause the muscles to become weak and not work properly. The electrical impulses help to determine how well the muscles are working and if there is any damage. The test is usually done on the arms and legs, but it can also be done on other parts of the body. The test is usually done in a doctor's office or a hospital. It is a quick and easy way to diagnose myositis.

HOW IS MYOSITIS TREATED?

There is no cure for myositis, but treatment can help to reduce symptoms and improve quality of life. Treatment typically involves corticosteroids and immunosuppressants.

Corticosteroids: Corticosteroids are a type of medication that is often used to treat myositis. They work by reducing inflammation throughout the body. While they are typically very effective, they can also cause several side effects, including weight gain, acne, and mood swings. As a result, corticosteroids are usually only used for short-term treatment. If you are considering corticosteroids for myositis, be sure to discuss the risks and benefits with your doctor.

Immunosuppressants: Immunosuppressants are the cornerstone of myositis treatment. For people with this condition, these drugs help to quell the immune system's overactive response. This, in turn, can reduce inflammation and improve muscle function.

There are a variety of immunosuppressants available, and the most appropriate one for each person will depend on factors such as the severity of their myositis and their overall health. Some common immunosuppressants used to treat myositis include methotrexate, azathioprine, and cyclophosphamide.

In some cases, a combination of immunosuppressants may be used. While these drugs can be highly effective, they can also come with side effects such as an increased risk of infection and gastrointestinal problems. As such, it is important to work closely with a doctor to ensure that the benefits of treatment outweigh the risks.

In some cases, physical therapy may also be recommended to help maintain muscle strength and function.

A POTENTIAL 3-STEP PLAN FOR MANAGING MYOSITIS

If you or a loved one has been diagnosed with myositis, it's important to work with a doctor to develop a treatment plan. In addition to medical treatment, several lifestyle changes can help to manage myositis.

1. Eat a healthy diet: Eating a healthy diet is important for everyone, but it's especially important for people with myositis. A healthy diet can help to reduce inflammation and improve overall health.

There is no cure for myositis, but a healthy diet can help to manage the symptoms and improve quality of life. The goal of a myositis diet is to reduce inflammation and support muscle growth and repair. Foods that are rich in antioxidants, omega-3 fatty acids, and protein are especially beneficial. In addition, it's important to avoid processed foods, sugar, and saturated fat. By following a healthy diet, people with myositis can improve their overall health and well-being.

2. Get adequate rest: People with myositis often experience fatigue, which can be exacerbated by a lack of sleep. It is therefore crucial for people with the condition to get enough rest. Most adults need around eight hours of sleep per night. However, people with myositis may need more than this. Aim to get at least 8 hours of sleep each night.

If you find it difficult to get enough sleep, talk to your doctor about ways to improve your sleep hygiene. Several fatigue-management strategies can be useful for people with myositis. These include pacing yourself and taking regular breaks during the day.

3. Exercise regularly: Myositis is a condition that causes inflammation of the muscles. It can lead to muscle weakness and pain and can make everyday activities difficult. Exercise is an important part of managing myositis and improving overall health. It helps to reduce inflammation, improve muscle function, and boost overall health.

Talk to your doctor about an appropriate exercise plan for you. Regular exercise can help you stay active and independent. It can also help you manage your weight, reduce stress, and improve your sleep.

Myositis can be a difficult condition to manage, but with the right treatment plan, it's possible to live a full and healthy life. If you have myositis, be sure to work with your doctor to develop an individualized treatment plan that's right for you.

MANAGING MYOSITIS THROUGH DIET AND NUTRITION

Diet and nutrition play an important role in managing myositis. Eating a healthy diet can help to reduce inflammation, improve overall health, and boost energy levels.

Foods to Eat

There are no specific dietary recommendations for people with myositis. However, general healthy eating guidelines should be followed. These include eating plenty of fruits, vegetables, whole grains, lean protein, and anti-inflammatory foods.

Fruits: Fruits are an excellent source of vitamins, minerals, and antioxidants, which are essential for managing the symptoms of myositis. Berries, citrus fruits, and stone fruits are some of the best options to include in one's diet.

Each type of fruit provides different nutrients that can help to manage the symptoms of myositis. For example, berries are a good source of antioxidants, which can help to protect cells from damage. Citrus fruits are a good source of vitamin C, which is essential for immune system function.

Stone fruits, such as apricots and peaches, are a good source of vitamins A and E, which can help to reduce inflammation. Including a variety of fruits in one's diet is an excellent way to obtain the nutrients necessary for managing the symptoms of myositis.

Vegetables: Vegetables are a good source of vitamins, minerals, and antioxidants. Aim to eat a variety of vegetables, such as leafy greens, cruciferous vegetables, and sweet potatoes. These nutrient-dense foods may help to reduce inflammation and improve muscle function.

Whole grains: Manage your myositis by incorporating whole grains into your diet. Whole grain bread, cereals, and pasta can help to alleviate symptoms associated with the condition. The nutrients and fiber in whole grains help to reduce inflammation and promote a healthy digestive system. Choose products that are made with 100% whole wheat or another whole grain for the most benefit. Look for brands that are certified by the Whole Grains Council.

Lean protein: Chicken, fish, and tofu are all excellent sources of lean protein. They are also low in saturated fat and cholesterol, making them heart-healthy choices. In addition, these proteins are easy to digest and are less likely to cause inflammation. As a result, they are good options for people with myositis.

Anti-inflammatory foods: When it comes to managing myositis, diet can play an important role. Several anti-inflammatory foods can help to reduce symptoms and improve overall health. For example, omega-3-rich foods such as fish, nuts, and seeds are known to help fight inflammation. Other potent anti-inflammatories include ginger, turmeric, and garlic. Incorporating these foods into the diet can help to manage myositis and improve quality of life.

Water: It's also important to stay hydrated. People with myositis are at risk for dehydration due to medications' side effects and increased urination. Aim to drink 8-10 glasses of water each day.

Foods to Avoid

In addition, it's important to avoid processed foods, sugary drinks, and excessive alcohol consumption. These can all contribute to inflammation.

Processed foods: Processed foods are high in sugar, salt, and unhealthy fats. They can also contain additives and preservatives that can trigger inflammation. For these reasons, it's best to avoid processed foods when managing myositis.

Sugary drinks: Sugary drinks such as soda, juices, and energy drinks contain empty calories and can trigger inflammation. When managing myositis, it's best to stick to water, unsweetened tea, and coffee.

Alcohol: Alcohol is a known irritant and can contribute to inflammation. People with myositis should avoid excessive alcohol consumption.

Supplements: Finally, be sure to talk to your doctor about any supplements you're taking. Some supplements can interact with myositis medications and may not be safe for people with the condition.

Myositis is a chronic autoimmune disorder that can cause inflammation and muscle weakness. While there is no cure for the condition, symptoms can be managed through diet and lifestyle changes. By incorporating anti-inflammatory foods into the diet and avoiding processed foods and sugary drinks, people with myositis can help to reduce symptoms and improve their quality of life.

SAMPLE RECIPES

Baked Flounder

Ingredients:

- 1 lb. flounder, fileted
- 1/4 tsp. salt
- 1 cup halved red grapes
- 1 tbsp. extra-virgin olive oil
- 2 tbsp. parsley, chopped finely
- 1 tbsp. lemon juice
- 1 cup almonds, chopped and toasted
- freshly ground black pepper, to taste

Instructions:

1. Preheat the oven to 375°F.
2. Place fish on a sheet tray. Season with olive oil, salt, and pepper.
3. Combine the almonds, grapes, lemon juice, parsley, 1-1/2 tsp. of olive oil, 1/8 tsp of salt, and black pepper in a bowl.
4. Bake the fish for about 3 minutes.
5. Flip the fish and return to the oven.

6. Bake for another 3 minutes, or until the fish is starting to flake, while the center is still translucent. Don't overcook.
7. Serve immediately, topped with the grape mixture.

Salmon with Avocados and Brussels Sprout

Ingredients:

- 2 lbs. of salmon filet, divided into 4 pieces
- 1 tsp. ground cumin
- 1 tsp. onion powder
- 1 tsp. paprika powder
- 1/2 tsp. garlic powder
- 1 tsp. chili powder
- Himalayan sea salt
- black pepper, freshly ground

Avocado sauce:

- 2 chopped avocados
- 1 lime, squeezed for the juice
- 1 tbsp. extra-virgin olive oil
- 1 tbsp. fresh minced cilantro
- 1 diced small red onion
- 1 minced garlic clove
- Himalayan sea salt to taste

- black pepper, freshly ground

Brussels sprout:

- 3 lbs. of Brussels Sprout
- 1/2 cup raw honey
- 1/2 cup balsamic vinegar
- 1/2 cup melted coconut oil
- 1 cup dried cranberries
- Himalayan sea salt
- black pepper, freshly ground

Instructions:

To make the salmon and avocado sauce:

1. Combine cumin, onion, chili powder, garlic, and paprika seasoned with salt and pepper. Mix well before dry rubbing on the salmon.
2. Place the salmon in the fridge for 30 minutes.
3. Preheat the grill.
4. In a bowl, mash avocado until the texture becomes smooth. Pour in all the remaining ingredients and mix thoroughly.
5. Grill salmon for 5 minutes on each side or until cooked.
6. Drizzle avocado on cooked salmon.

To make the Brussel Sprout:

1. Preheat the oven to 375°F.
2. Mix Brussels Sprout with coconut oil. Season with salt and pepper.

3. Place vegetables on a baking sheet and roast for about 30 minutes.
4. In a separate pan, combine vinegar and honey.
5. Simmer in slow heat until it boils and thickens.
6. Drizzle them on top of the Brussels Sprouts.
7. Serve with the salmon.

Asian-Themed Macrobiotic Bowl

Ingredients:

- 2 cups cooked quinoa
- 4 carrots
- 1 package of smoked tofu
- 1 tbsp. nutritional yeast
- 2 tbsp. coconut aminos
- 4 tbsp. sunflower sprouts
- 2 tbsp. fermented vegetables
- 1 cup of shiitake mushrooms
- 1 avocado
- 2 tbsp. hemp seeds
- 2-3 cooked beets
- coconut oil cooking spray

Dressing:

- 2 tbsp. miso paste
- 1 tbsp. tahini
- 1 tbsp. olive oil
- 1/2 lime, juiced

- 3 tbsp. water

Instructions:

1. Roast the carrots in the oven at 400°F for 30-40 minutes.
2. Wash the vegetables, trim, and spray them with coconut oil.
3. Add them to the oven. When they are cooked, set them aside till you are ready to assemble the Buddha bowl.
4. Make the dressing by combining all of the ingredients in a medium-sized bowl. If the dressing appears lumpy, add more water.
5. To build the bowl, put the quinoa on the bottom and then arrange the vegetables on top.
6. Sprinkle the bowls with hemp seeds and drizzle the dressing over top.
7. Now serve and enjoy!

Chicken Salad

Ingredients:

- 1 small can of premium chunk chicken breast packed in water
- 1 stalk celery, large, finely chopped
- 1/4 cup reduced-fat mayonnaise
- 4 romaine leaves or red leaf lettuce, washed and trimmed
- 8 pcs. cherry tomatoes or 1 ripe tomato, quartered
- 1 cucumber, small and sliced thinly

Instructions:

1. Drain canned chicken and transfer to a bowl.
2. Put in celery and mayonnaise.
3. Mix lightly. Don't crush the chicken.
4. In a separate shallow bowl, place the lettuce neatly.
5. Add the chicken salad in the middle
6. Add tomatoes and cucumber slices to the plate.
7. Refrigerate before serving, cover with plastic wrap.

Baked Salmon

Ingredients:

- 2 salmon filets
- 6 cups of fresh spinach
- 2 tsp. coconut oil
- 1/4 tsp. turmeric
- lemon juice
- salt
- pepper

Instructions:

1. Preheat the oven to 400°F.
2. Line a baking dish with parchment paper.
3. Marinate salmon filets in lemon juice, coconut oil, turmeric, salt, and pepper.
4. Let it sit for a few minutes. This may also be done the night before to help the juices and flavor get into the salmon.

5. Once the oven is ready, bake salmon for 15 minutes.
6. Add spinach and cook until ready. Season with salt and pepper to taste.
7. Take salmon out of the oven and put spinach beside it.
8. Serve and enjoy.

Asian Zucchini Salad

Ingredients:

- 1 medium zucchini, sliced thinly into spirals
- 1/3 cup rice vinegar
- 3/4 cup avocado oil
- 1 cup sunflower seeds, shells removed
- 1 lb. cabbage, shredded
- 1 tsp. stevia drops
- 1 cup almonds, sliced

Instructions:

1. Cut the zucchini spirals into smaller parts. Set aside.
2. Put almonds, sunflower seeds, and cabbage in a large bowl. Combine the ingredients well.
3. Add zucchini to the mixture.
4. In a small bowl, mix vinegar, stevia, and oil using a whisk or fork.
5. Pour vinegar mixture all over the zucchini mixture. Toss well. Make sure everything is covered with the dressing.
6. Refrigerate for 2 hours before serving.

Low **FODMAP** Burger

Ingredients:

- 1-1/4 lbs. ground pork
- 1/4 tsp. allspice
- 1/2 tsp. salt
- 1/2 tsp. white pepper
- 1/2 tsp. ground nutmeg
- 1/2 tsp. caraway seeds
- 1/2 tsp. ground ginger

Instructions:

1. Preheat the grill then prepare the patty.
2. Using a small mixing bowl, stir together the salt, pepper, allspice, nutmeg, and ginger until fully combined.
3. Place the ground in a large mixing bowl and add the spice mixture.
4. Mix thoroughly until spices are evenly distributed to the pork.
5. Make round, flat burger patties using the palm of your hands.
6. Grill the patties and serve with gluten-free buns and mustard sauce.

Stir-Fried Cabbage and Apples

Ingredients:

- 1 shallot, thinly sliced

- 1/2 apple, cut into cubes
- 1/4 savoy cabbage, sliced thinly into strips
- 3–4 radishes, sliced thinly
- 1/2–1 tsp. coconut oil
- salt, to taste

Instructions:

1. Pour some coconut oil into a wok.
2. Add shallot and cook until translucent.
3. Add the cabbage, radish, and apples to the wok.
4. Stir-fry for about 5 minutes. Don't overcook.
5. Add salt to taste.
6. Serve while warm.

Asparagus and Greens Salad with Tahini and Poppy Seed Dressing

Ingredients:

- 10 to 12 asparagus stalks, washed well and sliced into ribbons
- 5 radishes, washed well, and sliced thinly
- 2 to 3 rainbow carrots, peeled and sliced thinly
- 1 handful wild spinach
- 1 small handful of microgreens, washed well
- 1 small handful of sunflower greens, washed well
- optional: few pieces of chive blossoms

For the dressing:

- 2 tbsp. tahini
- 1 tbsp. poppy seeds
- 1 tbsp. extra-virgin olive oil
- salt
- pepper

Instructions:

1. For the dressing, whisk ingredients together in a small bowl.
2. In a separate bowl, toss salad ingredients into the mixture.
3. Drizzle dressing on salad upon serving.

Stir-Fried Cabbage and Apples

Ingredients:

- 1 shallot, thinly sliced
- 1/2 apple, cut into cubes
- 1/4 savoy cabbage, sliced thinly into strips
- 3–4 radishes, sliced thinly
- 1/2–1 tsp. coconut oil
- salt, to taste

Instructions:

1. Pour some coconut oil into a wok.
2. Add shallot and cook until translucent.

3. Add the cabbage, radish, and apples to the wok.
4. Stir-fry for about 5 minutes. Don't overcook.
5. Add salt to taste.
6. Serve while warm.

Roasted Chicken Thighs

Ingredients:

- 1 tbsp. avocado oil
- 1 pinch Himalayan pink salt
- 4 chicken thighs with skin
- 1 tsp. Primal Palate super gyro seasoning

Instructions:

1. Pour avocado oil over a medium-sized oven-safe pot.
2. Sauté over medium heat for 2 to 3 minutes or until the skins begin to brown.
3. Place the chicken in a large skillet over medium-high heat. Sear for about 2 to 3 minutes for each side, starting with the skin side.
4. Season generously with salt and Primal Palate Super Gyro seasoning.
5. Place the chicken in an oven preheated to 350°F.
6. Bake for one hour while covered.
7. Serve and enjoy.

Arugula and Mushroom Salad

Ingredients:

- 5 oz. arugula washed
- 1 lb. fresh mushrooms
- 1/4 tsp. shoyu
- 1/2 red onion
- 1 tbsp. olive oil
- 1 tbsp. mirin

For tofu cheese:

- 1/8 cup umeboshi vinegar
- 1/2 firm tofu

Instructions:

1. In a bowl, add the rinsed tofu. Crumble and pour in vinegar.
2. In a separate bowl add shoyu, red onions, salt, olive oil, and mirin. 3. Mix to combine.
3. Add in the arugula and toss to combine with the dressing.
4. Serve and enjoy.

Cauliflower and Mushroom Bake

Ingredients:

- 3 cups cauliflower florets
- 1 cup fresh mushroom, chopped
- 1/2 cup red onion, chopped
- 1/3 cup green onion, chopped
- 2 tsp. apple cider vinegar

- 2 tsp. lemon juice
- 1/2 tsp. salt
- 1/4 tsp. pepper
- 1 tbsp. olive oil

Instructions:

1. Preheat the oven to 350°F. Lightly grease a baking pan.
2. Combine red onion, cauliflower, olive oil, mushroom, apple cider vinegar, lemon juice, salt, and pepper in a bowl. Mix well.
3. Pour the mixture into the greased baking pan.
4. Place inside the oven and bake for 45 minutes. Stir.
5. When vegetables are golden brown and tender, remove them from the oven.
6. Garnish with green onions. Serve and enjoy.

Fresh Asparagus Salad

Ingredients:

- 1/3 cup of hazelnuts
- 4 cups arugula
- 1 tsp. ground pepper
- 4 tsp. lemon juice
- 2 tbsp. sea salt
- virgin olive oil
- 2 lbs. asparagus

Instructions:

1. Preheat the oven to 400°F.
2. Place hazelnuts on a baking tray with parchment paper. Place in the oven for 7 minutes.
3. Transfer hazelnuts to a plate. Optionally, to remove the skins, wrap the nuts in a towel and rub them vigorously.
4. Chop hazelnuts coarsely.
5. Remove the hard ends of the asparagus.
6. Place the stalks on the baking sheet you've used for the hazelnuts. Sprinkle 1 tbsp. olive oil and 1/2 tsp. of salt.
7. Bake for 8 minutes.
8. In a mixing bowl, combine pepper, salt, olive oil, and lemon juice. Mix well.
9. Place the arugula in a medium bowl. Drizzle ½ of the dressing over the veggies. Toss until everything is well coated.
10. Place arugula onto a platter.
11. Arrange asparagus on top. Sprinkle peeled hazelnuts on top.

Detox Bowl

Ingredients:

- 1/2 cup onion, diced
- 1-1/2 tbsp. olive oil or coconut oil
- 1 tbsp. ginger, grated
- 1 tsp. whole mustard seeds
- 1 tsp. turmeric
- 1/2 tsp. cumin

- 1/2 tsp. coriander
- 1/2 tsp. curry powder, add more for taste
- 1 small red chili pepper, dried, crumbled (adjust quantity for preferred spice)
- 3/4 tsp. kosher salt
- 1/4 lentils, soaked overnight
- 1/2 cup buckwheat, toasted or brown basmati rice, soaked
- 1-1/2 cup water
- 1 cup vegetable broth
- 2 cups chopped vegetables, such as broccoli, carrot, cauliflower, celery, a fennel bulb, and parsnips
- 2 tbsp. cilantro or Italian parsley, chopped
- lemon or lime, squeezed
- 1 tomato, diced

Instructions:

1. Heat up oil in a medium pot over medium-high heat.
2. Saute onion for about 2-3 minutes.
3. Lower heat to medium and add ginger to saute for a few minutes, or until it's fragrant and the color turns golden.
4. Add salt, spices, and pepper according to your taste. Stir and leave to toast for a few more minutes.
5. Put lentils and buckwheat or rice, followed by water, broth, and the remaining vegetables. Bring to a boil and cover.
6. Reduce heat to low and leave to simmer for about 20 minutes. Check every now and then for doneness.
7. Leave to cook for 5-10 minutes more if needed.

8. For porridge-like consistency, pour in more veggie broth.
9. Upon serving, top with tomato and cilantro or parsley. Dash with salt, pepper, and a choice of citrus. Drizzle olive oil if desired.

LIVING WITH MYOSITIS

Myositis can be a difficult condition to manage. In addition to dietary changes, several other lifestyle changes can help to reduce symptoms and improve quality of life.

Exercise: Exercise is an important part of managing myositis. It helps to maintain muscle strength and flexibility, and can also reduce inflammation. People with myositis should aim to get at least 30 minutes of moderate exercise each day. Consult with a doctor before starting an exercise program.

Stress management: Stress can trigger myositis flares and worsen symptoms. As a result, it's important to manage stress levels. There are several ways to do this, including yoga, meditation, and deep breathing exercises. In addition, talking to a therapist can help to identify and manage sources of stress.

Get enough sleep: Sleep is essential for overall health and can help to reduce inflammation. People with myositis should aim to get at least 7-8 hours of sleep each night.

Myositis is a chronic autoimmune disorder that can cause inflammation and muscle weakness. While there is no cure for the condition, symptoms can be managed through diet, lifestyle changes, and medications. By making some simple changes, people with myositis can help to reduce symptoms and improve their quality of life.

Conclusion

Myositis is a rare autoimmune disease that causes inflammation of the muscles. The three most common types of myositis are dermatomyositis, polymyositis, and inclusion body myositis.

The cause of myositis is unknown, but it is thought to be triggered by a combination of genetic and environmental factors. Symptoms of the condition can vary but may include muscle weakness, fatigue, and a rash.

There is no cure for myositis, but symptoms can be managed through diet, lifestyle changes, and medications. Some simple dietary changes that may help to reduce symptoms include incorporating anti-inflammatory foods into the diet and avoiding processed foods and sugary drinks. In addition, exercise, stress management, and getting enough sleep can also help to improve quality of life.

If you have myositis, it's important to partner with a healthcare team that can help you manage the condition. This team may include your primary care doctor, a rheumatologist, and a physical therapist. With the right treatment plan, people with myositis can lead active and fulfilling lives.

References

Articles. (n.d.). Cedars-Sinai. Retrieved September 22, 2022, from https://www.cedars-sinai.org/health-library/diseases-and-conditions/m/myositis.html.

Myocarditis—Symptoms and Causes. (n.d.). Mayo Clinic. Retrieved September 22, 2022, from https://www.mayoclinic.org/diseases-conditions/myocarditis/symptoms-causes/syc-20352539.

Myositis (Dermatomyositis, Polymyositis) - Symptoms, Causes & Treatments. Symptoms, Causes & Treatments | Arthritis Society Canada. (n.d.). Retrieved September 22, 2022, from https://arthritis.ca/about-arthritis/arthritis-types-(a-z)/types/myositis-(dermatomyositis,-polymyositis).

Myositis: Causes, Diagnosis, and Treatment. (n.d.). Hospital for Special Surgery. Retrieved September 22, 2022, from https://www.hss.edu/conditions_inflammatory-muscle-disorders-diagnosis-treatment.asp.

Myositis. (n.d.). [Text]. Retrieved September 22, 2022, from https://medlineplus.gov/myositis.html.

Nutrition Tips for People with Myositis | HSS Myositis Center. (n.d.). Hospital for Special Surgery. Retrieved

September 22, 2022, from https://www.hss.edu/conditions_nutrition-and-myositis.asp.